INTERMITTENT FASTING FOR VEGANS

A healthy and effective guide for vegans to loss fat with intermittent fasting

Contents

If you feel you have appreciated my effort, I kindly ask you to leave a (positive) review! It will help me to create something new and useful for your interest: =)

M.T.

CHAPTER ONE: BASICS OF THE INTERMITTENT FASTING VEGAN DIET

If you've never followed a vegan diet before, you may not be familiar with what it entails and the principles behind it. In essence, a vegan diet avoids all animal products in lieu of foods derived from fruits, vegetables, seeds, nuts, grains, and other nutrients from the earth.

Reasons People Choose a Vegan Diet

Vegan diets are popular today for a host of reasons:

- Veganism does not harm animals.
- Eating plant-based foods is better for the environment and the planet.
- Vegans typically spend less at the grocery store.
- You can grow your own primary food sources as a vegan.
- A vegan diet may help reverse or lessen the effects of certain conditions and may provide relief from some digestive ailments.
- Many people lose weight and report having more energy when practicing veganism.

Foods Not Permitted on a Vegan Diet

It may surprise you to learn that, in addition to meat, poultry, and fish, there are other foods not allowed on a vegan diet. These include all dairy products, eggs, and even honey for most vegans. In this way, veganism is different from vegetarianism, which does permit dairy, eggs, and honey.

Vegans believe that these animal products are not beneficial or necessary for the body, and many think they are also unethical because of the way animals are treated in their production. The simple act of removing honey from a beehive, for example, disturbs the bees, disrupts their habitat, and deprives them of a winter food source.

Foods Encouraged on a Vegan Diet

Fortunately, the earth provides vegan dieters with an enormous range of foods they can eat. Typical vegan meals are composed of vegetables, fruits, legumes, and the like to provide flavor, variety, and nutritive value. Popular vegan staples include:

- seeds, nuts, and nut butter
- tofu, seitan, and tempeh
- plant-based milk and yogurts
- algae and seaweed
- fermented and sprouted foods
- grains and cereals
- legumes (beans and peas)
- fruits and vegetables

There are various versions of the vegan diet that further define eating habits for different personal needs. Some vegans enjoy eating only raw foods, which means nothing is cooked over 118 degrees

Fahrenheit. A variation on this diet is eating raw foods until around four o'clock in the afternoon, after which time a regular cooked vegan meal can be consumed. Other vegan subcategories include eating mainly starches and eating mostly low-fat plant-based foods.

History and Culture of Veganism

It is unknown how long people have been practicing intentional veganism, but it is thought to go back to the very early Hinduism. People of the Hindu faith, to this day, do not eat meat. There are other references to abstaining from animal products throughout history, including in the Book of Genesis in the Bible.

Modern veganism began in the mid 19th Century in England and has gathered an enormous following since then. Once labeled a 'hippie' diet from the 1960s, veganism is now a way of life for many, whether it's because they wish to avoid exploiting animals or simply like how much better they feel when avoiding animal products on the dining room table.

The Science Behind the Vegan Diet

The vegan diet has been studied exhaustively by the medical community, seeing it as a possible cure for diseases that commonly plague society. In addition to lowering the risk of certain types of cancer, heart disease, and diabetes, a vegan diet can reduce arthritis symptoms and lower obesity. A recent study by Oxford University maintains that eating a vegan diet could cut roughly eight million deaths per year, both by improving personal nutrition and by reducing greenhouse emissions caused by raising livestock for food.

Far from being a fad diet without scientific support, veganism comes recommended by researchers and nutritionists, and its benefits far outweigh any inconveniences experienced.

Chapter Summary

Key takeaways from this chapter are:
- The vegan diet means eating *no* animal products, including eggs, dairy, and honey.
- There are lots of great plant-based options to provide flavor and nutrition to a vegan diet.
- A vegan diet is practiced for a variety of reasons, including health benefits and animal treatment ethics.
- Veganism is practiced for thousands of years, and it is scientifically well studied.

CHAPTER TWO: WHERE VEGANS GET NUTRIENTS

Vegan diets that contain a range of natural foods, lots of fruits and vegetables, and a minimum of processed foods provide plenty of vitamins and minerals. However, one of the biggest concerns for vegan dieters is getting enough protein since animal products, which are typically high-protein sources, are not consumed. Let's take a look at some top vegan protein sources and why they are so important to your nutrition.

How Much Protein Do You Need?

In spite of the popularity of high-protein diets these days, the average person doesn't need to eat a ton of protein to stay healthy and active. It is recommended to eat about 0.36 grams of protein for every pound you weigh, and slightly more is suggested for vegans because of the nature of plant proteins--about 0.41 grams per pound of weight. That works out to about 51 grams of protein per day for a 125-pound person or 74 grams of protein for someone weighing 180 pounds.

How do you know how much protein you are consuming? Packaged foods contain the amount of protein per serving on the label, so you just need to carefully calculate your serving at a time to calculate the protein included. When preparing raw, bulk, or unpackaged foods at home, simply use a nutritionist's food chart to call your groceries.

What Is Protein Anyway?

Proteins are compounds found in nature and are made up of long chains of amino acids (nature's building blocks). You need protein to maintain muscles and to keep your hair, nails, and skin healthy. If you're an athlete, still growing, or a pregnant woman, your protein needs may be higher than those of others because of greater demands on the body.

There are 20 different amino acids that can be combined to form proteins, but nine of them should be taken from your diet. These are commonly called 'essential amino acids.'

Types of Protein

Without these essential amino acids, a protein is not considered 'complete'; that is, it won't be as effective in helping you stay healthy and energized.

Meat and eggs are complete proteins in and of themselves. So are quinoa, soy, and buckwheat. However, many plant-based foods are not complete proteins. How do vegans get around this and ensure they get enough complete protein every day? By combining foods to get the right mix of amino acids, thereby creating complete proteins.

Vegan Sources of Protein

It's actually easy to get complete proteins while on a vegan diet because the foods that combine to make them tend to go well together. Classic examples of vegan complete protein combos include:

- hummus and pita bread

- rice and beans

- grains or nuts added to spirulina (a member of the algae family)

- peanut butter on wheat bread

- lentils and corn or lentils and barley (such as in soup or chili)

Other sources of protein that are ideal for incorporating into a vegan diet are:

- chia seeds

- hemp seeds

- pumpkin seeds

- Ezekiel bread

- seitan, tofu, and tempeh

- nuts and nut butter

- veggie burgers and hotdogs

- soy or other veggie crumbles

Are you worried that all this protein combining is starting to sound too complicated? Many vegans find that if they eat a wide variety of foods every day, they don't really need to worry about combining proteins in a formal way because it happens naturally through their food selection. In general, if you eat the foods on the lists above, you should find you are getting adequate protein. One way to check is to keep a log for a week or so to see that you have enough diversity in your vegan diet.

Vegan Substitutions

One aspect of vegan dieting that some people find challenging is not replacing meat at meals but eliminating animal products in other places, like dairy and eggs in baking or recipe ingredients. In addition to vegan cheeses made from nuts, you can use things like applesauce, chia seeds, tofu, mashed banana, ground flaxseed, and arrowroot powder in your baked goods and casseroles.

Chapter Summary

This chapter discussed how to incorporate protein into a vegan diet without eating animal products. Important points to remember include:

● Protein is a necessary dietary component for your body's optimum function.

● There are different types of protein, and it's desirable to eat complete proteins as a regular part of your diet.

● You don't need to eat animal products to get plenty of protein in your diet.

● There are tons of protein sources available to vegans that taste great.

CHAPTER THREE: WHAT IS INTERMITTENT FASTING?

You have probably heard of fasting, which is abstaining from food. You may have had to fast before surgery or blood tests at the doctor's office. Some people also fast for religious reasons. Intermittent fasting is going without eating for a set period of time at regular intervals; hence, you fast intermittently. Unlike most diets that are concerned with *what* you eat, intermittent fasting is all about *when* you eat. You'll read why that's so important in the next chapter.

Intermittent fasting is embraced for a number of reasons, some of which will be discussed in subsequent chapters. One of the most popular motivations for intermittent fasting is weight loss, although intermittent fasting can also be done to help with various health issues, to feel less bogged down by food, and even to live longer.

Different Types of Intermittent Fasting

Just like with the vegan diet, there are subtle variations within intermittent fasting too. One common intermittent fasting schedule is known as '16:8' because you fast for 16 hours and then eat within an eight-hour window every day. Another top intermittent fasting plan is the '5:2' diet, which entails eating normally for five days out of the week and then radically restricting calories to about 500 per day for two days per week. Some people fast every other day, alternating with eating normally on other days.

One of the most appealing aspects of intermittent fasting, as you have probably noticed, is that it can be adjusted to meet your personal needs. In addition to a rotating day type of fasting plan, you can also fast every day and manipulate your eating window to best work with your unique schedule. If you're an early riser, you may want to have your first meal by 10 am, eat between 10 and 6 pm, and then fast from 6 pm until 10 am. But if you're more of a night owl, you can start eating at noon and push your fast off until 8 pm.

Chapter Summary

Here are the most important things to remember about intermittent fasting.

- Intermittent fasting is the practice of going without food at regular intervals.
- You can fast intermittently every day, every other day, or a few times per week.
- Intermittent fasting has lots of compelling reasons for its current popularity, especially the ease of starting and flexibility.

Keep reading because the next chapter is all about the health benefits of intermittent fasting.

CHAPTER FOUR: HEALTH BENEFITS OF INTERMITTENT FASTING

Intermittent fasting has been well studied by doctors and dietitians and found to have numerous health benefits. But before you learn about all those advantages, it's important to understand exactly how intermittent fasting works.

The Effects of Intermittent Fasting on the Body

When you eat any sugars that your body doesn't use right away, they are stored in your cells as fat. Insulin, a hormone produced by the body to help it use sugar properly, is the freight train that carries sugar to the cells for storage. When you eat all day long, especially a diet high in carbohydrates, your insulin keeps getting spiked, causing you not only to gain weight but to eventually lose sensitivity to insulin itself.

Whenever your insulin levels go down, the body recognizes there's no immediate sugar to be used as fuel, so it releases fat from where it has been stored in the cells to give you energy. One way to induce your insulin levels to decline naturally is to stop eating. This helps you lose weight by burning fat.

Fasting is a reliable way to repeatedly reduce insulin in your bloodstream. If you fast regularly, over time, your body becomes better at regulating and using insulin, known as improving insulin sensitivity.

What Else Can Intermittent Fasting Do?

While people have been fasting for centuries, including intermittent fasting (whether accidentally or intentionally), this method of eating didn't come under the scrutiny of medical researchers until the 1930s. Doctors at Cornell University discovered that rats that ate less lived longer. Fifteen years later, researchers at the University of Chicago revealed that alternate-day feeding had the same effect.

More recent studies on animal models have demonstrated that intermittent fasting can slow down or protect participants from:

- damage from strokes
- Alzheimer's disease
- Parkinson's disease
- cognitive decline

Why Intermittent Fasting Is So Successful Now

Let's go back to the basics of intermittent fasting for a moment to see why this way of eating is so popular today. Obesity and diabetes/pre-diabetes are an epidemic in the Western world, particularly in the United States. A well-studied dietary regimen that allows people to improve their sensitivity to insulin, prevent diabetes, reduce the severity of diabetes, and lose weight as intermittent fasting does, makes sense.

Many people have lost the ability to know when they really need to eat. Intermittent fasting restores that by at first restricting your eating hours and then by helping the body's hormones tell you when it needs fuel. People who follow intermittent fasting programs report no longer being hungry all day long, reduced unnecessary snacking, and a return of normal hunger pangs only when they should eat (more on this in Chapter Twelve).

Chapter Summary

This was an important chapter, so take a moment to revisit the health benefits.

Intermittent fasting:

- Lets you burn fat when you're not eating.

- It can help stabilize insulin and prevent the progression of diabetes.

- Helps the body return to normal hunger cues.

- In animal models shows far-ranging benefits related to brain function and longevity.

The next chapter in this book discusses even more health benefits of intermittent fasting and how it can even have a healing effect on the body.

CHAPTER FIVE: HEALING POWERS OF INTERMITTENT FASTING

In Chapter Four, you learned about the health benefits of intermittent fasting. But did you know there are even more advantages to this eating plan that may involve healing the body?

A Review of Insulin and Intermittent Fasting

You just read about how intermittent fasting helps your body use and respond to insulin more subtly, but it's worth repeating here when discussing the healing powers of intermittent fasting. Improving insulin sensitivity doesn't just help you lose weight, which can be a great benefit on its own; it can prevent prediabetes from progressing to full-blown diabetes. In some cases, intermittent fasting can even reduce the severity of Type 2 diabetes when practiced under the care of a physician. Those healing effects alone make intermittent fasting worth considering for many people.

Inflammatory Healing with Intermittent Fasting

Increasing insulin sensitivity is just the proverbial tip of the iceberg when it comes to the physiological healing that's possible with intermittent fasting. One of the other great benefits of this eating regimen is its ability to ease inflammation for some people. Studies on intermittent fasting show it can reduce inflammatory markers--biological signs that show up in blood tests--for a range of inflammation, including arthritis and even asthma symptoms.

Why is healing inflammation so important? Not only does reducing inflammation potentially alleviate pain, but it also reduces the risk of high blood pressure and cardiac disease. Intermittent fasting is doubly helpful with regard to blood pressure because it can decrease inflammation and, at the same time, directly lower blood pressure as well.

Digestion and Intermittent Fasting

One place in the body where many people experience inflammation, often without even knowing it, is in the digestive system. We have both beneficial and not-so-helpful bacteria (flora) in our gut that can fall out of balance with the wrong diet and by constant eating. Some flora may even work their way into the bloodstream through microscopic tears in the digestive tract (known as 'leaky gut syndrome').

Intermittent fasting allows the gut flora to rebalance itself because you're not constantly filling the digestive tract with food and asking it to work. Normal digestive enzymes, hormones, and other chemical compounds can finally settle into a more natural state.

Other Healing Benefits of Intermittent Fasting

The ability of the body to rest when not eating cannot be underestimated with intermittent fasting. When you eat, you not only stress your digestive system but your entire body. Blood is shunted from other areas of the body to the stomach and intestines to process food. (Remember the old adage about not swimming right after eating? That's why.) Sleep may be disrupted if you're trying to digest food too late at night. Vital cells that are needed for healing are slowed down to make way for digestion.

It's good to give your body a break from constantly trying to process food. Think of it like shutting down the assembly line in a factory to allow the machinery to cool off and prevent wear and tear. This is especially true if your body requires serious healing for a condition or injury, such as recent surgery, a sports trauma, or a serious bout of the flu.

This also holds true for chronic illnesses, like thyroid disease, adrenal insufficiency, and fibromyalgia. You may find that once you have practiced intermittent fasting for a while, the symptoms of long-term conditions improve, and you have more energy because your body is not being over tasked with too many functions.

Chapter Summary

In this chapter, we looked at the healing powers of intermittent fasting.

- Intermittent fasting can help reduce inflammation, which not only relieves pain but may benefit long-term cardiovascular health.
- It can also reduce gut inflammation and help restore digestive health.
- Intermittent fasting also gives your body a break from processing food so it can devote its energy to other functions.

CHAPTER SIX: PILLARS OF INTERMITTENT FASTING

Here are some key points that have been touched on and for which you will receive gentle reminders throughout the rest of the book, the 'rules' of intermittent fasting if you will.

1. Choose an intermittent fasting schedule that you can realistically sustain. You may think fasting for 20 hours per day will help you achieve results faster, but if you can't do this for more than a few days, you will only wind up quitting before you see any benefits. Instead, pick a plan that works for your schedule and ramp-up to your desired fasting time by incrementally reducing your eating window (see Chapter Ten).

2. Do not eat anything during the time you are supposed to be fasting. You are allowed to drink as much water, tea, black coffee, and diet soda as you like during your fast times. Stay hydrated by quenching your thirst with water and herbal tea. If possible, avoid diet soda, which some studies show may make you want to pig out when you do finally get to eat.

3. Do not overeat when your fast time is up. Technically, you consume as much food as you love while you're not fasting, but gorging will have multiple negative effects. If you are trying to lose weight, eating too many calories, even with

fasting, may keep you from dropping pounds. Also, overeating taxes your digestive system, which is one of the things you are trying to avoid with intermittent fasting.

4. Spread your eating out over your non-fasting window, especially if you are fasting for a portion of every day. While you can fast for most of the day and eat one meal per day, you may feel less cranky and have more energy if you eat several times within your eating window. As mentioned above, you don't want to overeat with intermittent fasting, and eating only once per day may unwittingly encourage that.

5. Eat a range of vegan foods when you are not fasting, so you are sure to get the protein, vitamins, and minerals you need. Avoid junk food, even if it doesn't contain animal products.

6. You may have questions that only your personal healthcare provider can answer.

7. Stop fasting or reduce your fasting time if you experience any of the following:
    - light-headedness
    - dizziness
    - fainting spells
    - nausea
    - blurred vision

- weakness

- extreme fatigue

- inability to sleep

<u>*Chapter Summary*</u>

This chapter reviewed the 'rules' for intermittent fasting. Go over them a few times before you start to make sure you understand how to fast.

- Pick a realistic schedule for fasting.

- Don't eat food during your fasting window.

- Don't overeat during your designated eating times.

- Know the signs that tell you to slow down or reduce your fasting time.

CHAPTER SEVEN: COMBINING VEGANISM AND INTERMITTENT FASTING

Mixing a vegan diet and intermittent fasting sounds like a giant task, but it's really quite a fantastic pairing if you approach it right. This chapter will give you some tips for combining the two.

Advantages of Veganism During Intermittent Fasting

One of the biggest challenges faced by anyone doing intermittent fasting is hunger pangs. That hunger will rear its angry head faster if the food you consume during your eating window is digested quickly.

Fortunately, natural vegan food (not vegan junk food--yes, there is such a thing!) is generally high in fiber, whether you're eating legumes, vegetables, or fruits. So, one big key to feeling full longer is to keep eating lots of fiber and to eat it throughout the periods when you are allowed to eat.

Other foods that are vegan staples also help keep your stomach from grumbling. Fats take longer to digest than carbohydrates, so be sure to add some to your diet.

Foods to Stay Satiated

If you're heading to the grocery store and want to purchase some foods that make you feel satiated, here's a great list to start with:

- legumes (beans, lentils, peas, chickpeas, etc.)
- leafy greens (lettuce, spinach, kale, etc.)
- cruciferous veggies (broccoli, cauliflower, etc.)

- fruits and vegetables with the peel intact (apples, peppers, pears, etc.)
- nuts, nut butter, and seeds
- olives and olive oil
- avocados
- squash and pumpkin
- berries and fruits/vegetables with seeds (pomegranates, cucumbers, etc.)
- fibrous vegetables (celery, asparagus, green beans, etc.)
- whole grains and whole-grain products (pasta, cereal, bread)
- dried fruits and raisins
- hemp products
- dates and figs
- veggie burgers and veggie crumbles
- vegan 'cheese' made from nuts
- edamame (soybeans)

Chapter Summary

Combining a vegan diet with intermittent fasting is easy and natural.
- Eat high-fiber foods, which are staples of the vegan kitchen, to stay feeling full longer.
- High-fat vegan foods also keep you feeling satiated.

In the next chapter, you will learn some advice on starting a new diet.

CHAPTER EIGHT: HOW, WHEN AND WHERE TO START

The beauty of a vegan intermittent fasting regimen is you can start virtually anywhere, any time. There are a few tips. However, that will make commencing your new eating plan go much more smoothly.

Go at Your Own Pace

If you are starting both a vegan diet and intermittent fasting at the same time, you may feel overwhelmed with so much change happening at once. Instead, before trying intermittent fasting, try the vegan diet for a few weeks or so.

If you are going from being a full-on carnivore to vegan, you may want to take even more time. Start by weaving meatless meals into your weekly menu. Then, stop eating meat, fish, and poultry. Finally, eliminate other animal products like dairy and eggs to complete the transition.

Likewise, you can ramp up your intermittent fasting schedule, so it's not a total shock to your body all at once (see Chapter Ten). Let's say you've decided to follow a plan that allows for eight hours of eating, followed by 16 hours of fasting. You may be ravenous when you first start fasting, to the point where you give up on the diet before you have a chance to reap its benefits. Rather than psyching yourself out, try fasting for 10 hours first, then 12, then 14, and finally 16.

Take a Look at Your Calendar

While you can certainly start a vegan intermittent fasting plan today if you like, you may want to check your calendar first to make sure it's the ideal time to increase your chances for success. If you are heading to a wedding on the coming weekend, taking a vacation with the family, or running your first marathon, it may not be the time to utterly revamp your diet. Look for a time when life is relatively calm, so you won't have any hurdles that make the change next to impossible.

Map Out a Plan of Action

Whenever you start a new eating regimen, you want to have a plan in place before you begin. Think of it as a roadmap to a new destination when driving your car.

Take a realistic look at your daily schedule to decide when it's best to fast and when it's best to eat. Build-in cooking prep time, so you won't sabotage yourself with junk food or resort to grabbing a burger when you're starving.

Enlist a Support Team

Making big dietary changes is challenging. Be aware that some people will be enthusiastic cheerleaders for you, while others may resent your foray into better health. Ignore the naysayers, and focus on people who will support you in your endeavor.

There are lots of places to find people who will aid you in your new eating adventure or even join you in intermittent vegan fasting:

- the gym or health club

- running, cycling, and triathlon training groups
- the office or workplace
- online chat groups and forums
- organic and health food stores
- local produce growers, community-supported agriculture, and farmer's markets
- vegan restaurants
- cooking groups and courses
- organizations and clubs where you are a member

Chapter Summary

Starting intermittent fasting as a vegan is simple, especially if you know a few top tips for success.

- Plan well in advance and pick a low-stress time to start.
- Get support for your efforts and tune out naysayers.
- Break your new life change into manageable chunks as needed; start by going vegan first, then add intermittent fasting.

CHAPTER NINE: EXERCISE AND WORKING OUT WHILE FASTING

One prevalent questions from newbie intermittent fasters are, "How do I exercise or work out while I'm fasting?" Surprisingly, many people actually have more energy and feel better when they fast, so working out isn't an issue. But if you're someone who is concerned about "bonking" during your workout, read on to learn some suggestions for keeping your energy up.

Timing Your Workouts

One of the biggest worries when exercising in combination with intermittent fasting is how to time your workouts. In many ways, the answer is a personal one that depends on your metabolism, your unique body chemistry, and the type and intensity of exercise you perform.

Most athletes have to experiment a bit to find a schedule that works best for them. In general, if you're not working out hard, you have more leeway in timing your exercise sessions. Light exercise means less demand on the muscles and less competition between the digestive system and the musculoskeletal system.

If you up the intensity of your sport, however, you will likely need to give more thought to when to exercise in relation to eating. If you are trying to lose weight through exercise and fasting, it's best if you can exercise right before eating at the end of a fasting period, as long as you can do it without losing your energy. Exercise gives your metabolism a boost for a few hours afterward, so when you reward yourself with a post-workout meal, your body is still in calorie-burning mode. This schedule is ideal for morning exercisers.

However, if you can't make it through a workout without feeling fatigued, or if lack of stamina is affecting the quality of your performance, you may need to exercise during an eating window or within a few hours of eating. Are you an evening exerciser? This schedule may work better for you. Also, try to split up your eating, so you're not exercising after one huge meal.

Nutritional Needs and Exercise

The intensity of your exercise, coupled with your own physiology, determines how much and what type of food you need to eat to stoke your body's engines when working out. Also, your desire to lose or maintain weight figures into your menu.

As you've already learned, a vegan diet can provide plenty of protein as well as food that keeps you full all day. You may want to go up a bit on the protein if you're training super hard, such as for a marathon or triathlon, or if you are trying to increase muscle mass (muscle is built on protein). You also want to eat as well-rounded a diet as possible, so you get all the nutrients you need. If you feel you are missing vitamins and minerals from your diet, you can add over-the-counter supplements to fill in.

Exercising and Losing Weight While Fasting

One of the boons of intermittent fasting is that you can lose weight fairly easily without limiting calories, simply by observing your fasting schedule and not overeating during your food windows. While weight loss is enhanced by exercise, even when practicing intermittent fasting, know that you can ease up a bit on the workouts if you are already losing weight through fasting. Instead of forcing yourself to do exhausting cardio for hours, you can enjoy other forms of exercise for fitness, like:

- tai chi or soft martial arts
- dancing
- softball
- swimming
- walking or light jogging
- Pilates
- yoga
- recreational cycling
- golfing
- light resistance work
- gardening and housework

Additional Tips for Working Out and Intermittent Fasting

Working out while practicing intermittent fasting should be fun and rewarding. Once you figure out the perfect schedule for you, use these tips for improved performance:

1. Stay hydrated. Drinking plenty of water throughout the day will help you to feel full and make you less likely to cheat by eating when you shouldn't. Water is essential to keep your muscles and joints functioning at an optimum level. And water also helps your body remove toxins and waste through the urinary and digestive systems. You'll process and absorb nutrients better when you're thoroughly hydrated.

2. Try a little caffeine before working out. A small amount of caffeine, such as the amount in a cup of black coffee, taken a right before exercise can increase the uptake of free fatty acids in the bloodstream. What does that mean? Caffeine can help you burn fat instead of glycogen (sugar-based fuel) during exercise.

3. Has some food prepped for immediately after exercise if that's when you're scheduled to eat? Particularly if you are making recipes from scratch at home, you need to do a little work in advance to make sure you have healthy foods available to you. Take a cooked sweet potato, a container of berries, or a handful of nuts with you to the gym if you have a long ride home after working out. Otherwise, you may succumb to the temptation of junk food when you're starving and pressed for time.

4. If you're worried you're not getting enough nutrients for your workout routine, consult your physician or a professional dietician or trainer experienced with vegan diets and intermittent fasting.

5. If you feel the need for a cardio burn, but don't want to devote an hour or more every day to running or similar exercise, try HIIT or high-intensity interval training. HIIT typically entails doing short bursts of aerobic exercise, interspersed with recovery periods, for about 30 minutes. Many fans of intermittent fasting report HIIT suits them very well and adds a bit of oomph to their weight loss efforts.

Chapter Summary

Exercising or working out can be combined with intermittent fasting, but it just takes a little thought, and sometimes trial and error, to make it work for you.

• Find the right time to exercise based on your unique needs and to eat schedule.

• Make sure you are eating healthy vegan foods to meet all your nutritional needs.

- Because you may already be losing weight with intermittent fasting, you can usually lighten up on the cardio workouts and have fun with other types of exercise for strength and flexibility.
- Prepare in advance: have water and healthy foods ready at all times.
- A little caffeine consumed before exercise can help you burn fat instead of glycogen. Fat is a more efficient source of fuel; save the glycogen for your brain!

The next chapter gets into the nuts and bolts of intermittent fasting by offering you a sample fasting plan; you can start as soon as now.

CHAPTER TEN: SIMPLE FASTING PLAN

Do you need a little more help getting started with an intermittent fasting plan? Here is a plan to begin fasting that starts out easy and ramps up gradually over the course of three to four weeks to a longer fasting window. Don't forget; it's perfectly fine to go at your own pace. If you're not ready for a longer fast, stay where you are for a bit longer.

An Intermittent Fasting Plan You Can Start Today (16:8 Fasting)

Week One:

- Eat between 7 am and 7 pm (12 hours)
- Fast between 7 pm and 7 am (12 hours)

This schedule of 12 hours on/12 hours off gets you used to eating within set times and starts getting you into the mindset of fasting, so you're paying more attention to when you eat and your body's hunger cues. You'll notice that it capitalizes on your circadian rhythm (your body's natural timetable that revolves around sunrise and sunset). Additionally, this plan gives you a few hours after your last meal before bed. Numerous studies demonstrate that eating too close to sleep increases the risk of diabetes and obesity.

If you work nights or swing shifts, you will obviously have to adjust this fasting plan, but if you normally work during the day, it's best if you can take advantage of your body's natural fasting time during sleep at night.

Week Two:
- Eat between 8 am and 6 pm (10 hours)
- Fast between 6 pm and 8 am (14 hours)

You'll note that this week, you're adding two hours to your fast time.

Week Three:
- Eat between 10 am and 6 pm (8 hours)
- Fast between 6 pm and 10 am (16 hours)

The third week of your intermittent fasting plan adds another two hours to your fast window. You have now reached the 16:8 daily fasting schedule. Even though you are technically fasting for 16 hours per day, about seven or eight hours of that time is spent sleeping, so a good chunk of your abstinence from food will pass quickly.

If this schedule doesn't work with your job, exercise, family, or social schedules, simply adjust it. You can still fast for 16 hours by eating from 11 am until 7 pm, for example. Just make sure the ratio of eating to fasting time stays the same.

- Eat between 12 noon and 6 pm (6 hours)
- Fast between 6 pm and 12 noon (18 hours)

Fasting for 18 hours may be more than most people can handle, and it's definitely something you need to work up to slowly. But the extra fast time can benefit people who want to lose weight by intermittent fasting. If you try the Week Four schedule and find it's too much for you, go back to Week Three and stay there.

Alternative Fasting Plans

Here are two fasting plans for people who don't want to fast every day. Maybe you know yourself well enough to know that you won't stick to a daily plan. The best intermittent fasting plan is the one you can stay with long term and fashion into a lifestyle!

Alternative Plan #1 (5:2 Fasting):

- Eat normally, consuming a healthy vegan diet on Monday, Wednesday, Thursday, Saturday, and Sunday.
- Fast on Tuesday and Friday, eating no more than 500 calories on each of those days.

You'll see this plan doesn't involve any mandatory times for completely going without food, other than when you're sleeping. However, if you eat one or two small meals that total 500 calories within a small window of time, your fasting days will be similar to the fasting windows observed during the 16:8 plan reached by Week Three above.

You can shift this schedule to any 5:2 ratio during the week. Just make sure that your two fasting days are non-consecutive days of the week (not two days in a row). You can actually eat quite a lot of food on a vegan diet and still only consume 500 calories. The foods below are easy to eat in small portions and can be prepared to give you adequate vitamins and protein.

Suggested foods for your 500-calorie days include:

- vegan yogurt
- hummus and vegetables
- legume soup
- salads
- cereal and grains
- nuts

Alternative Plan #2 (Alternate-Day Fasting):

- Eat normally on Monday, Wednesday, Friday, Sunday.
- Fast on Tuesday, Thursday, and Saturday.

This plan will create a rolling schedule, where one week you are fasting on Tuesday, Thursday, and Saturday, and the next week you are fasting on opposite days. The idea is to constantly alternate your fast days with your normal eating days. Some people like to eat nothing on their fast days. But most people find this very difficult, so they eat 500 calories on their fast days.

Chapter Summary

You can start intermittent fasting today with any of the plans outlined above.

● Plan #1, the most common, lets you eat for eight hours per day, and then you fast for 16 hours. This plan is practiced every day of the week.

● Plan #2 lets you normally eat for five days of the week, and you fast on two days by eating only 500 calories per day. This is the best plan for people whose family or social lives revolve around meals or for whom daily fasting may be challenging.

● Plan #3 is an alternate-day fasting schedule, where you normally eat on one day and eat only 500 calories the next.

The next chapter will outline an exercise plan to go with your intermittent fasting diet.

CHAPTER ELEVEN: SAMPLE WORKOUT PLAN

Are you wondering how to integrate your exercise regimen with intermittent fasting? Have you been a bit of a couch potato recently and want to get back to working out when you start your intermittent fasting plan?

Here is a sample workout plan you can begin right away. Remember from previous chapters that if your main goal with intermittent fasting is to lose weight, you may do that with fasting alone. It's better to combine diet and exercise for weight loss and overall health, but you can cut back on the cardio a little with intermittent fasting and enjoy other types of exercise that aren't so exhausting and hard on the body.

Weekly Exercise Plan

Monday:

- 30 - 50 minutes brisk walking or light jogging
- 5 minutes of crunches and/or planks
- 5 minutes cool down with gentle stretching

Tuesday:

- 20 - 30 minutes HIIT (high-intensity interval training) workout
- 10 minutes cool down with gentle stretching

Wednesday:

- 30 - 60 minutes of any low-impact exercise for joint mobility and flexibility: yoga, Pilates, tai chi, light water exercise/swimming
- (Optional: take this day off if you want two days of rest per week.)

Thursday:
- 30 - 90 minutes of playing a sport: tennis, softball, soccer, fencing, horseback riding, skating, basketball, canoeing, dancing, etc.
- 10 minutes cool down with gentle stretching

Friday:
- 20 - 30 minutes HIIT (high-intensity interval training) workout
- 10 minutes cool down with gentle stretching

Saturday:
- 30 - 60 minutes of any low-impact exercise for joint mobility and flexibility: yoga, Pilates, tai chi, water exercise/swimming

Sunday:
- Day off--no exercise

What's the theory behind this exercise routine? You'll notice it varies high-intensity work with stretching, moderate activity, and sports. This allows your body to recover after heavy workouts.

The variety makes the plan interesting, so you don't get bored doing the same thing day after day. Switching things up keeps your body guessing, too, so you're more likely to burn calories with every workout instead of plateauing. By doing a range of different types of exercise, you build strength, maintain cardiovascular health, improve your range of motion, and develop both fine and gross motor skills. You can obviously change this routine to suit your hobbies and schedule, but if you're at a loss or need some structure, it gives you a place to start. The idea is to alternate heavier and lighter workouts, both in terms of intensity and time, and include some fun, like playing on a team or trying a new sport.

Chapter Summary

While you can lose weight with intermittent fasting alone, it's better to combine it with exercise for overall health and fitness.

- Because intermittent fasting is already helping you burn calories, you can cut some of the cardio workout time from your schedule if you are doing it nearly every day.
- Vary your exercise routines in terms of intensity and time. Alternate heavy workouts with ones that include more stretching and gentle exercise.
- Include a day of fun sport for variety and skill-building.

The next chapter will discuss what you can expect when you start intermittent fasting, including both the benefits and challenges you are likely to encounter.

CHAPTER TWELVE: WHAT TO EXPECT AND POTENTIAL EFFECTS

Here's a look at some issues intermittent fasters commonly face as well as tips for getting over initial hurdles. Of course, there are also great benefits, so you'll be reminded of those too, lest you forget why you want to make changes to your eating habits.

Adjusting Your Schedule

For most people starting an intermittent fasting regimen, changing their schedule is one of the most challenging aspects. You will likely be adjusting the times you eat, which may mean giving up breakfast with the family or going out for late-night dinners with friends. If you lean towards frequent social eating or those family meals are crucial for you, 5:2 fasting or alternate-day fasting are probably best for you. You can get your fasting in and still have days where you can keep your social schedule intact.

Don't forget to look at your sleep schedule too. Especially in the beginning, you may find you need more snooze time than normal, and even once you have acclimated to the diet, you want to make sure you get enough rest. Fasting is a minor, manageable stress on the body, but it can become overwhelming if you are unduly fatigued.

You've already read about possibly needing to adjust your workout schedule too. It's likely you'll need to experiment with a few different eat-fast-exercise configurations to figure out which one works best for you.

Dealing with Hunger Pangs

Another common hurdle new intermittent fasters face is managing hunger. You will feel hungry at times at the start of your new fasting lifestyle, but that usually goes away for the most part. Even so, you will realize that being a little hungry isn't a catastrophe. If you tough it out for a little while, ghrelin (your hunger hormone) recedes on its own.

Sometimes you can confuse hunger with thirst. You may find your 'hunger pangs' abate when you quench your thirst.

Eating Strategically

Strategic eating is another way to manage hunger. If you have an eight-hour window in which to eat and you only eat one meal, guess what? You will probably be hungry during part of your fasting time. But if you spread your meals out over the entire eight-hour window, you'll be less likely to experience hunger, and you won't run out of energy at work or during exercise.

Enjoying Desirable Results

You just read about how ghrelin, the hormone that tells you you're hungry, comes and goes over time. One of the benefits of intermittent fasting is that your ghrelin sensitivity, in addition to your reaction to insulin, becomes more acute. After practicing intermittent fasting for a month or two, you'll probably notice you're not getting as hungry as you used to. Congratulations, your body is returning to its normal, natural way of being!

You've read about the benefits of intermittent fasting in previous chapters, but let's review them again as inspiration for when you're first starting out:

- lowers cholesterol
- lowers insulin level in the blood
- improves insulin sensitivity
- promotes weight loss
- reduces inflammatory markers
- helps rebalance gut flora
- decreases the risk of various brain conditions and cognitive decline
- lowers blood pressure

Chapter Summary

This chapter focused on what to expect when you begin intermittent fasting.

- Expect to have some hunger pangs initially, but they will get better.
- You will have to adjust your schedule somewhat to eat fewer hours of the day.
- Intermittent fasting offers so many wonderful benefits; you will likely find they outweigh any negative issues.

If you feel you have appreciated my effort, I kindly ask you to leave a (positive) review! It will help me to create something new and useful for your interest: =)

M.T.

CHAPTER THIRTEEN: FINAL CONSIDERATIONS

Before you head off to try the intermittent fasting and a vegan diet on your own, there are a few final things to consider and a few reminders worth mentioning.

Weight-Loss Maintenance on Intermittent Fasting

If you begin intermittent fasting with the goal of losing weight, you may reach your goal but not desire to drop any more pounds. You want to be careful that you don't fast too much and lose weight you can't afford to part with.

Some people's weight naturally levels off without an adjustment to their intermittent fasting diet. However, if you are worried about continuing to lose after you hit your goal weight, here are a few tips:

• You don't want to go overboard or resort to eating junk food. But an extra avocado, a little more olive oil on your salad, or an extra sweet potato here and there may be just what you need to stop losing and stay at your desired weight.

• Look at your exercise plan. Are you still working out like you need to drop 20 pounds even after you've lost the weight? You should either keep working out hard and increase your caloric input or cut back a little on the exercise. If you're doing a lot of high-intensity or cardio exercise, consider swapping out some hard training days for something more gentle, like yoga, tai chi, or walking.

● Adjust your fasting plan. Some people eat in only a tiny four-hour window for drastic weight loss, but this may not be sustainable once you hit your goal weight. Try lengthening your eating period by an hour or two.

Intermittent Fasting Is Not a Miracle

Intermittent fasting has changed people's lives for the better, whether by improving health conditions or simply making them feel more energetic. However, fasting is not a solution to every health problem, nor does it produce overnight results. You need to first make sure you don't have unrealistic expectations, and you need to give intermittent fasting at least a month of religious practice to see if it works for you. You may feel better right away, but you may also need more time to see anti-inflammatory results, to better regulate your insulin sensitivity, and to restore your normal cues for hunger.

A vegan diet is also not a miracle worker. While eating plant-based foods is a wonderful choice for your overall health, you still can't gorge on whatever you like (an entire pan of vegan brownies) or eat only vegan junk food. Likewise, when eating between fasts with intermittent fasting, you shouldn't be overeating. Moderation in all things related to diet is definitely the way to go.

You Should Not Feel Sick While Fasting

Some people feel better almost immediately when they begin an intermittent fasting plan. However, other people feel tired, cranky, hungry, and generally out of sorts even after a few weeks in. If you find yourself feeling this way, it doesn't necessarily mean intermittent fasting is wrong for you; it could mean you need to tweak your personal program for your individual needs:

• Examine the length of time you are fasting. It could be too long for you. Try shortening your fast time by an hour or two to see if you feel better.

• Your fast window may be fine in terms of length, but you may need to shift it to earlier or later in the day to accommodate your schedule and nutritional needs.

• You may have selected the wrong fasting plan for yourself. For example, you may be practicing daily 16:8 fasting when 5:2 or alternate-day fasting might work better. Try switching plans to see if that has an effect on your mood and health.

• Are you consuming food throughout your entire eating window, or are you stuffing all your eating into one meal? While a few people do well with only eating one meal a day, most people feel better when they can spread their eating out. Try eating two or three smaller meals during your non-fast times to keep up your energy and stave off hunger.

• If you are an exerciser, especially one who trains hard, you may need to adjust your workout time to better suit your new intermittent fasting plan. You may also need to time your meals differently with your workouts.

• Are you eating high-quality vegan foods? Getting enough protein and other nutrients? Be sure to review the chapters on vegan dieting to see if you can improve your sources of nutrition. Also, even with a healthy diet of natural foods, it's possible to miss some nutrients. Potassium, for example, is a difficult element to consume insufficient quality through diet alone. You may need a supplement to pick up the slack.

• Don't forget to stay hydrated! Water will help you digest your food and absorb nutrients better and will keep you feeling full longer.

• Are you cheating? Remember, you can only have black coffee, tea, water, or diet soda during your fasts. Nothing else is allowed. Intermittent fasting can't work if you aren't actually fasting!

Contraindications for Intermittent Fasting

If you have doubts about fasting, consult your healthcare provider first. Even though intermittent fasting can mitigate many of the symptoms of diabetes, anyone with Type 2 diabetes should check with a doctor first before trying to fast (and Type 1 diabetics who are insulin-dependent should never fast; see below).

If you belong to any of the following categories, you should not fast:

- children
- underweight people
- malnourished people
- people with a history of eating disorders
- people with chronic hypoglycemia (without physician's consent)
- Type 1 diabetics (and possibly Type 2, depending on doctor's advice)
- pregnant women
- lactating women
- people who need to take medicine throughout the day with food
- people under chronic stress
- individuals suffering from hormone dysregulation (e.g., menopause or hypothyroidism) without regulating hormones first
- anyone who has had a serious negative reaction to fasting in the past

You Can Do It!

Making any big changes in life can be scary and require us to create a different version of ourselves to succeed. But without change, we stagnate and never reach the goals we aspire to, including having a healthier body. Be confident you can change your life. You will find that taking that one step towards improving your diet and wellness will have a ripple effect, and you will be able to then handle other challenges you have been aspiring towards. Onward!

<u>*Chapter Summary*</u>

Now you have new insight into both the vegan diet and intermittent fasting, and it's time to try it yourself.

• Review the contraindications for intermittent fasting, and make sure it's right for you.

• Be realistic about your goals, and give the planned time to work.

• Be flexible, and be ready to make adjustments to an intermittent fasting lifestyle to suit your personal needs.

• Use small tweaks to adjust your intermittent fasting plan if you are using fasting to lose weight and don't want to keep losing after you hit that magic number on the scale.

• Have confidence in your ability to change, and not only will you improve your health, but you'll also open the door to reaching other life goals you've always wanted to achieve!

CHAPTER FOURTEEN: TASTE AND INTERMITTENT FASTING

This is one of the primary concerns for every newbie, but it must be resolved during this week of preparation. It is how we are affected by taste and how we must protect our sense of taste.

Taste is not originally meant only for pleasure. Taste is meant to be able to pick out the foods you need that can provide the nutrition your body requires.

Taste translates to appetite, and appetite dictates what food you eat. When your body needs a certain nutrient, it gives you the appetite to look for and consume that dish that contains that nutrient. If you are a lifelong vegan, that's not a problem, but if you are new to veganism, you are going to have an appetite for things that are not on your menu.

Here is how that works:

When you are a kid, your parents introduce you to food that is part of your culture and upbringing. If you are English, you get Bangers and Mash for breakfast; if you're Mexican, you get Tortillas and Quesadillas, and if you are American, you get cereal and toast. That's what you grow up with (I know it's a lot more than that - it's just an illustration).

When you consume the array of foods you are given, your body records and associates different foods with different experiences and with different nutrition, so, for instance, if you had sunflower seeds in the morning with your cereal, your body will record all the nutrition it received from ingesting that recipe - Vitamin E from the sunflower seeds, being one.

From that point, whenever your body runs low on Vitamin E, it is subconsciously going to make you have an appetite for sunflower seeds. It gives you the appetite by the taste of the sunflower seeds and the association it makes in your brain between the need for Vitamin E and the taste of sunflower seed.

Taste is very important in our ability to keep ourselves healthy and to replenish what we need when we need it. It is important to safeguard the foods we eat and not get complacent with highly flavored foods. When you get started on a lifestyle of intermittent fasting, you will find your taste buds are heightened, and you have the appetite for foods you need rather than the ones you are addicted to.

That's what this week will help you do. It will help to signal to your mind that the foods it craves habitually are no longer available. That way, by the time you get to your first fasting week, you've primed your mind and body into relying on taste as your guiding tool to pick out foods you need.

What does that do for you? Well, it saves you from eating unnecessary calories and putting on unnecessary weight. It works like this. If I am craving Vitamin E from sunflower seeds, but instead of choosing natural sunflower seeds, I choose the one that is processed and salted, here is what happens. The salt appeals to my taste, and that creates a habit, but the processed seeds have lower Vitamin E, and so to get the Vitamin E I need, I take more seeds to satisfy the deficiency. That results in higher caloric intake, and that gives me the extra weight I don't need.

So, when you get off the seasoning, and the flavoring and your tastes can accurately choose the food that is the source of the nutrient it needs, then you choose the most natural foods you can find during this preparation week, and by the time you get to your initiation week, your palate will be cleansed, and your appetite will accurately reflect what your body needs to replenish.

Remember, Intermittent Fasting is a lifestyle change; we will have to get used to it. That's why you cannot think of this as a diet and something you will do for a week then get back to your old lifestyle. This is a change to the fundamental way you see yourself and understand your senses. It is a fundamental way you make use of your natural fat-burning cycle. It is the natural way the human body thrives.

Foods to Rethink

There isn't any particular food group you need to rethink, but the ones that you must keep an eye on are the prepared foods that come heavy with flavorings. Stay away from those at all costs. Flavorings will mess with your sense of taste, and the effect cascades into your choice of food and your frequency of consumption.

If you eat a healthy meal, not only will you not feel hungry in a few hours, you can go for a day or two without needing to top up your fuel reserve. If you find you cannot stay away from the flavor, then all the more reason you must do this.

So, the foods to rethink are the ones that come with flavorings, like the prepackaged chips and dips, seasonings and garnishing, snacks that are heavily flavored. The easy way to categorize them is to be wary of all prepackaged and processed foods. If you must consider it, it's probably something you should avoid.

Once you take care of that and you clean your palate, then enjoy all the fruits, nuts, vegetables, and seeds you can get your hands on. I do not consume mock meats and mock milk - you know, the ones made from soy or other non-animal sources but try to mimic the taste of dairy and meat - that's what you are trying to avoid - flavorings.

The key to a successful Intermittent Fasting lifestyle is to change two things about your approach to food. The first is to take away the habitual element of food - and in this case, we are talking about the food you eat for taste instead of nutrition. The second is to change the way your taste buds are employed. If you use your taste buds to pick the food your body needs, you will find you to increase your health and vitality.

In your prep week, there are a few things you must accomplish. The first thing is you must reflect on the food you are consuming and the reasons you are consuming it. Having fun food is not dangerous, as long as you can sufficiently keep it from distracting your body from making the correct food choices based on taste. As a vegan, you have minimized most issues, but by taking on this new lifestyle, you will further eradicate the confusion your taste senses must contend with.

There is such a thing as healthy snacks. If you think there aren't, then it's a mindset problem. The world around you wants you to think junk food has all the pleasure of eating. That's not true. Fruits and veggies in the correct mix with herbs and spices in the correct quantities are pleasing and healthy. If you eat what your body needs, the pleasure is more than you get from eating junk food - and it is good for you. That is one benefit of Intermittent Fasting; you will start to hear your body's needs more clearly, and when you give it what it needs, the pleasure you get from food is more than you get from the junk chemically-flavor-ridden foods.

That's one thing most food enthusiasts do not realize. Food can be a pleasurable experience when you eat intermittently and give the body what it is looking for. Eating just for habit is missing the most important ingredient of the meal: a need for it.

Once you get through preparation week by shunning all the extra flavors and addictive substances, and you make advances in cleaning your palate, you are almost ready to get started with Initiation week, which starts with Zero Day (don't worry; these concepts will be explained later). Ideally, if you can go away with this, it will be great. If you can take the weekend off, go to the mountains, or go to the beach, go away with someone you know who will support you on this, or go away alone, then you will make Zero Day that much more effective.

Overview of Initiation Week

Initiation week is the week you start to feel the effects of the full program. It comes after a week of preparation, and it is manageable when you are prepared for it, rather than jumping in the cold. In initiation week, there are days when you will eat, and there are days when you will fast totally, only consuming water.

The seven days should start at the point you complete your dinner on the last day of your preparation week. And that is the start of your Zero Day. Zero-Day is 36 hours and should span three days and two nights. It is specifically designed to initiate you into a new lifestyle, so be mentally prepared to undertake this. All the forces of your mind will convince you this is a bad idea. Unless your doctor tells you this program is not for you, there is no reason you shouldn't undertake it.

After the seventh day, it becomes a series of periods alternating between fasting and eating. You will see this will allow your body to utilize its metabolic pathways and allow you to have a better quality of life and a lesser incidence of food-related illnesses.

Your food revolution starts with the change in perspective over your place in this world and how you energize that existence. There are two stages to your intermittent fasting, and we will get to that in later chapters. For now, let's assume you are a fasting newbie. You have not ventured into the idea and the world of fasting. So, we will take this gently.

We will start with the basics of fasting and show you why Intermittent Fasting is not fasting and how you can align yourself with the forces and habits that will result in long-term health. Most of us associate the word fasting with starving, but luckily, with intermittent fasting, this isn't the case.

The only thing you must consider is removing heavily processed foods. That's your biggest enemy. It's not the fats or the natural sugars or the caffeine or the vegetables. As long as the food is natural, you're ok. Processed foods add many things that do not do your body good. So, switch out of the processed foods and head to the farmer's market and shop the organic aisle. As a vegan, you are probably already doing so.

Once you have that in place, we are ready to start.

Intermittent Fasting is not about starving yourself. It's about changing the schedule of your meals to a more natural one. If you can get rid of the habit of regular eating, you will realize your body doesn't need to take in lots of food on a schedule. Even the way it stores and uses those stores changes when you stop feeding it every four hours. Your body starts to be smart and act like it naturally should.

CHAPTER FIFTEEN: ZERO DAY - 0 TO 36 HOURS

The object of the first day is to go through thirty-six hours free from consuming any food. This will show you those feelings of doom and despair you feel when you fast are just in your mind. You will come out of the 36-hour period still alive and feeling better than you felt before going in.

Zero-day aids in the removal of toxins that have accumulated, and it resets your body's natural eating schedule. You'll be surprised to see the body feels very agile, and your mind is very sharp due to extinguishing and removing toxins from your body.

Even when regularly eating outside the fasting period and the food is not as nutritious as it can be, like say with processed food with high levels of toxins, the body is actually working overtime to remove these toxins. You don't feel it until you get to a point where you get sick, then you start to feel it. Until then, your body is actually working hard. The first thirty-six hours in your intermittent fast will help your body catch up and remove the toxins and prepare your body for its new lifestyle.

This first thirty-six hour is also crucial because it is one of the make-or-break events in your fasting lifestyle. If you have a mindset that the fasting process was unpleasant, then you will automatically create a frame of mind that you will always have towards fasting - this is precisely why you want to create the environment for a good experience by going away for Zero Day.

For those of you who worry it is impossible for the human body to go without food for 36 hours, I assure you, and you can check this with your physician, this is not the case. Your body can easily handle it because it has enough stores of fat and nutrition to sustain and replenish you, so don't worry unless you're diabetic, have a metabolic disease, or you have an illness; then you may have a problem, so you must check with your doctor.

Once you've checked with your doctor and if he says you're healthy to do it, the only impediment to intermittent fasting is in your head, and that's what you must remove in these thirty-six hours. You must focus on living your life outside your head in these 36 hours, starting on Zero-day because if you recoil within your head, you will have doubts and hardships.

Remember, your body has been used to consuming at least three meals a day - it's a habit no different from smoking; it's no different from having caffeinated drinks because your body has created a habit.

Your mind will rebel, so be prepared for that. The first thirty-six hours shows you how much your mind can put up a fight, but not to worry; nothing's going to happen. You will get an insight into how your mind works and how it creates excuses when you do not feed a habit.

At this stage, you will learn:

1. The list of excuses your mind makes to execute a habit
2. The feeling you have when you do not perform a habit
3. The way your body changes from burning food to burning fat

Actually, intermittent fasting can act as a way of meditation. You will examine your mind and its habits almost as an external observer. I have learned to control my mind better in other habits and negative behaviors.

You can do it for 36 hours. You can fast for seven to ten days straight if you want to. I have fasted for nine days straight with only water, and the feeling is amazing when you come out of it. I do this once in six months, besides the intermittent fasting lifestyle I already have.

The reason we started with a thirty-six hour fast is that the first twelve hours was not fasting. In the first twelve hours, you still have remnants of your last meal within you, and that is slowly metabolizing into energy, and your body's absorbing it, so the first twelve hours don't count, so you should start right after dinner. Let's say you have a sensible dinner around 7. Don't eat what you normally eat for dinner or worry about the next thirty-six hours.

Once you finish that meal, and you have a glass of water, that's it. You're done. Nothing else should pass your lips, except water, for the next 36 hours.

Importance of Water

When you are on a diet, especially when doing the Intermittent Fast, you must hydrate your body adequately and frequently drink to flush the system. With this in mind, consume no less than 2 liters per day for a regular lifestyle or 3 liters per day if you work out heavily. I keep two liters of filtered water ready and near me at all times. Having ordinary activities of daily living, like have a heavy game of racquetball or a heavy gym session, then the water I consume after the game doesn't count for the total amount I consume for the day.

The thing about water is it is the best liquid to keep you hydrated. Fasting does not mean any water. Fasting means you drink more water. There are two reasons you drink more water when you fast. One: remember, your body is trying to rid itself of toxins, and the more fluid circulating, the easier your body gets to flush these toxins out. So, the more liquid you have in you, the more efficient your immune system becomes because your circulatory system becomes more efficient. Two: it also helps you quell your hunger as it fills your stomach, and you will feel fuller.

Keep your required ration of water for the day in bottles and keep the bottles on the counter. This will make it more visible and difficult to forget how much water you have had and how much more you must drink. (Maybe one or two can be in the fridge for cool water, but most should be room temperature.) When the water is too cold or too warm, it changes your metabolism. So, keep the water at room temperature. And then you just go through bottle after bottle until your daily ration is done. One healthy morning habit is to put a pinch of sea salt in a large bottle of water, and you should have it as the first thing in your morning.

First 36 Hours

So, you start day zero with total water fast. In water fast, the idea is to cleanse your system and change your mind's habit of food consumption. It will also conclusively show you that you do not need to eat constantly to survive.

Have a glass of water at room temperature as soon as you are out of your bed. Don't drink ice-cold water, and don't drink it warm either. The idea is to not shock the system in the morning.

At the end of the thirty-six hours, actually just one day, you have only fasted for twelve hours because the other twenty-four hours went by while you were asleep. So, if you think about it, you start after dinner on the first day, and soon after that, you get to bed; you sleep until morning, and let's say you wake up at seven in the morning; the first twelve hours have gone. Now, you will go to 7 pm, which is a second twelve hours, which is when you are supposed to have your next dinner, but you don't, and you've also skipped lunch and breakfast that day. That's only 12 hours of not eating. Soon after your last dinner time, you go to bed. Now that brings us to your next twelve-hour period. When you wake up, it's 7 am, and you have done 36 hours. It doesn't seem like much, but you have just placed your body on a healthy track.

Post 36 Hours

When your first 36 hours are done, you must break the fast gently. You can't have a heavy meal right after fasting. You will get severe cramps and stomach aches. Your post-fast meal should be something you can gently introduce to your stomach and something that will help you with altering your metabolic pathway. Remember, you're burning fat now for fuel, and you want to reintroduce your metabolism to burn calories from the intake.

One of the major things about Intermittent Fasting is to get you to shift from relying on food in your belly to relying on the fat stores. To do this, you want to lay off the sources of sugar and carbohydrates. This is not exactly the Atkins diet, and it's not like the Paleo diet either. What you are doing is retraining your body to use the energy it needs from the excess stores in your body.

A better way to understand the food you should consume is based on what you feel like eating and how much, but your body is not ready to tell you this information yet. Because you are still running on habit, at this point, anything your body tells you it wants, you should consider it suspect. When you get to the second stage, you can feel what you should have for your next meal, but for now, you must bring in the discipline to counter false signals your mind is sending you.

The first meal after 36 hours will be breakfast. This should be your lightest meal of the day, and it gets your system up and running. Salads, nuts, tofu, and broth are good options for your first meal. If you can throw in some seeds or almond milk, that would be good too because one opportunity of fasting is rebalancing the bacteria population in your gut. By cleansing your stomach and rebalancing good bacteria, you will have a better rate of absorption of your food, so you get higher doses of nutrients for the same calories.

When you get on Intermittent Fasting, one thing you should think about is that there is a balance you must keep between calories and nutrients. The higher amount of nutrients you get for the least number of calories you take in allows you to keep a healthier body frame. It also allows you to build muscle mass rather than fat mass.

But for now, you want to keep your food intake to supply nutrients more than you need calories (just remember you can get a zero-calorie diet without fasting. Anything you eat has calories. Even if you chew and swallow paper, it will give you calories).

The best place for nutrients and low calories is steel-cut oats. It has only 300 calories per cup yet contains zinc, selenium, manganese, and phosphorus. It also contains polyphenols. One cup of oats without sugar for lunch, after your 36-hour fast, will get your body the nutrients it needs after the first day, without the extra calories, which you don't need.

CHAPTER SIXTEEN: 36 HOURS TO 48 HOURS

Day Three - 37th Hour to 48th Hour

You are now on your third day of the Induction Week of your Intermittent Fast. You are still very much alive, and you are in no danger of starving (you never were). What is bothering you and casting shadows of doom is just your mind. It will do everything to make you search for food. This mechanism has guaranteed our survival as a species. The ones that didn't search for food after fasting didn't survive.

You should be able to do some workouts, and you must be able to get some dopamine racing through your brain. For this, hit the gym with cardio workouts and lift heavyweights. Lifting heavy weights with full compound movements will make sure that, during fast, you will not lose your muscle mass due to atrophy. The workout should also kickstart your metabolic pathway.

Whatever water you drink at this point does not count toward your daily quota of 2 liters. Notice that nowhere here do we mention the possibility of you being hungry. Hunger is just a sensation - and that is the sensation you must learn to deal with. Your body is in no danger.

The one important chemical change that has happened is that you will have low insulin levels. This will promote the burning of fat much faster. Your meals should be whatever you feel like eating but without the additional artificial flavors. The point of the artificial flavor is to trick your taste buds into craving more food.

The main thing now is for you not to have a meal at the regular times. Forego the regular lunchtime meal and instead have a low carb - high nutrition snack with plenty of protein. Granola bars are a great way to treat your stomach. I typically have no-sugar granola with unsweetened almond milk for my meal of the day. Since it's hard to find granola bars that are healthy, I suggest you make your own. Here is a recipe that works well:

Snack Recipe 1

Use two cups of oats, 1 ½ ounce of raw sunflower seeds, 3 ounces of coarsely crushed almonds, ½ a cup of wheat germ, some vanilla extract, 10 ounces of dried fruits of your choice - apricots, raisins, dried cranberries, cherries, and blueberries. Warm a skillet and add a tablespoon of freshly pressed sunflower oil, and put in the sunflower seeds and almonds. Allow them to cook for a while, then add the oats. Once warm, add the dried fruits and the vanilla extract. Stir it, so it doesn't stick too much to the pan. A little sticking is ok.

Lay it out on the tin foil. Fold the tin foil over it and roll it to the thickness you like. Open the foil and fold the mix. Cover with foil and roll again. Do this a few times for a dense bar. Then put it in the fridge. You can have this as a snack once or twice a day on the days you are not fasting.

For the rest of the day, you really should eat whatever you feel like - without artificial flavoring or processed foods.

Remember, this is just for the induction week. Once you get to the regular week, it's never going to be this complicated. It will be straight-forward, and you can eat everything you want as long as it is healthy for you.

At this point, your food cravings would have reduced, and you are not as hungry as you thought you would be.

Timewise, you are at your 48th hour - the end of your third day. Remember, you started on Friday, and you fasted all Saturday. You broke fast on Sunday, and you've eaten all day when you felt hungry. It's now Sunday night, and you are getting ready to fast, starting after dinner and going all the way to Tuesday morning.

The second half of the Week

The Fourth Day - 49th hour to 84th hour

The fourth day is not as hard as the first or the second, and you get into the rhythm of things. The fourth day is when you fast for another 36 hours. Work out that evening before you start the fast and have an increased metabolism that night when you get to bed. You will burn more than the 600 calories you did the night after the oats or other meal you consumed.

Again, you consume nothing more than water. No less than 2 liters per day, not including any water you drink during or right after a workout. Try to work out on the morning of the fourth day as well to keep your body at peak metabolism. Remember to take a pinch of sea salt with the water you consume.

One thing that may happen to many people on the fourth day is that they have a dry mouth. So, drinking water actually becomes a necessity more than a rule. If you have a dry mouth, don't worry about it. As long as you generally feel healthy, you are urinating regularly, and your urine is clear, you are doing great. If your urine turns dark yellow, you are drinking way too little water.

This 36-hour fast brings you to the fifth day. You're almost at the end of the Induction Week, and you have carried yourself far. Be proud of yourself. Check on your blood pressure and your energy levels. Make sure you are still making it to the gym and that you are keeping your daily work and family routine.

The idea is to weave a new habit into an existing schedule and displace the old habit. Your lunch hour at work should be spent at the park or the beach. Don't follow your friends to the cafe or accompany them for food. It's not going to help. Get fresh air, and if you like, go to the gym at lunch. It will give you a boost for the second half of the day.

You are on the home stretch, and your body is getting used to switching between its metabolic pathway. You should start to feel more energy, and at the same time, you will feel more clarity and drive. Hold on to that feeling.

You will be surprised how the body has been dependent on the act of eating and on the taste and pleasure of food, so it has actually forgotten to do anything else, and it has actually forgotten that it need not eat daily. Food has become your porn - an addiction and like any addiction, and the best way to get away from it is to stand up to it. Your body will follow.

Congratulations, you are coming to Day Six!

Day Six - 85th Hour to 96th Hour

On the eve of Day Six, you should prepare for your next 36-hour fast. Begin with the resolve that comes from the confidence that, no matter how difficult it was, you've made it this far. Reflect on the path you have taken. Appreciate your accomplishment.

You can eat anything you wish in the next 12-hour window if it is not flavored and it is made of clean, non-processed foods. The taste should come from the ingredients you use in your cooking, not from sweeteners and flavor crystals. At this point, you can also have an increased sense of taste, and it is easier for you to taste all the ingredients in the food.

Don't indulge in anything sweet, except for fruit, and only ones that have a high glycemic index. Fruits with a high glycemic index prevent your insulin levels to peak, which usually leads to hunger and binge eating.

Bring fruits back to your diet and eat anything you want as long as you are not overly full. Have nothing that has been processed or has corn syrup and added sugar. My best sixth-day menu includes whole wheat pasta in olive oil with miso and avocado paste. You can try to taste the pure olive oil to see how well-developed your taste is after fasting. Before I did intermittent fasting, I usually couldn't taste the difference between olive oils. Now I can.

For breakfast, add a few spoons of lemon juice to your morning water portion and bananas as they have important minerals you'll need.

One of the important aspects of induction week is to break the dependence on your scheduled meals. You are a free person, and you should not be subjected to scheduled meals that control your life. Feed your body when it needs food, not when it is convenient for someone else. Eat only when you must and never eat for pleasure - in time, a new pleasure will come from eating fresh, clean, natural food.

Last Day

Good work coming this far! For the final day, repeat what you did on your fasting day, but remember you will go to bed with oatmeal as your pre-fasting day meal. And then go to bed and follow 36 hours of fast for your last day.

This introductory week is all most people need to get their systems realigned. In this week, these are the things you accomplished, whether you realize it or not:

1.Less dependency on scheduled meals
2.Less dependency on habits.

3.Altered perspective of food as a source of nutrition, instead of it being a source of pleasure

4.At least a 10-pound weight loss (depending on your initial body weight)

5.Achieved mind over the body

6.Acquainted yourself to eat-light-feel-light

The next chapter will get you ready to talk about what is going on with your body and what you must do to keep this up as you move forward. Intermittent fasting is not to make you suffer. It is about making you realize you can do without the regular and systematic introduction of food. The problem most people face is they are so addicted to the pleasure of food and the habit of eating that fasting becomes a mystery to them.

It's not fasting. It's just giving your body enough food, so it can use what it needs to replace its nutritional usage and provide itself energy to go through the day. It's also about activating both forms of metabolism in your body and following an eating rhythm your body has evolved during thousands of years.

When you fast, you should come to the realization you spend so much time and energy, and resources on food, thinking of food, traveling to get food, and whatever else we do that relates to food that we have allowed it to take over our lives. Intermittent fasting will not only allow you to lose the extra weight and feel better about yourself, but you will awaken one morning and feel like you can take on the world.

CHAPTER SEVENTEEN: INTERMITTENT FASTING LIFESTYLE

What you have seen so far is the Intermittent Fasting Induction Week, designed to change your body and act as the buffer between your old lifestyle and you're new. You can't go from what you have been practicing daily for the last ten, twenty, thirty, or more years and expect to have your body be all right with it. That's the purpose of the induction week. It introduces your body to intermittent fasting.

But now that you are done with induction week - what's next? Well, now you get started with your regular days. For your regular day, you have two options to choose from. One with strenuous workouts, and the other with light workouts. The choice you make depends on what your goals are - whether you are planning to sculpt your body or to have lots of energy and sharp focus.

Overview of Post Induction

The best way to have Intermittent fasting is to go through rapid cycles of feasting and fasting. While the induction week got you to explore and make use of your dormant metabolic pathway, this section will advance the switchover rate between your regular metabolism and your fat-burning metabolism.

If you are a marathon runner, you know what it feels like to switch over from regular metabolism (where you are burning calories from the food you just ate) to lean metabolism. It's what marathon runners call 'hitting the wall.' When you have calories in your belly, and you start the marathon, you get to a point where you deplete them, and you get to the point of exhaustion. The body takes the time to switch over and start burning fat, and you know the body is switching over because that is the time you feel like you can't go on and you want to stop. This is when you see athletes slow down, and you can see the immense pain in their faces. Then they get their second wind, and the energy comes back, and they pick-up and start running again.

Why the second wind?

Because their body just switched fuel sources. Most athletes train long hours, not only to build up their speed, strength, and efficiency but also to deduce the time they spend in the energy-less state when the body is switching over to burn fat. What we have done in the Induction Week is to bring online the ability to switch over. By doing the 36 hours on and 12 hours off Induction Week, you have been training your body to switch over quicker. As you get into the real week, and you increase the pace and the frequency to 18 on and six off, you will find your body will step up to the increased pace, and soon your switch-over rate will improve. When this happens, you will find that, as soon as you eat, the body will obediently source its energy from the food you have just consumed and rapidly switch over to fat-burning during the 18 hours you are fasting. It is an efficient system and one that will get you to peel off the weight, keep it off, and have an abundance of energy - and what is better is that, pretty soon, you will create a habit of the whole thing. This will make it easier for you to make it a lifestyle move rather than an unmotivated forced move.

Daily Switchover

In the daily switchover, you will be changing your entire routine, so you will focus only a fraction of your time on food, and the rest of your time would be spent on other productive activities.

This is the 16-8 daily split. That means you will fast 16 hours a day and then have an 8-hour window to eat. In that 8-hour window, you can taper the balance of your meals to reflect your lifestyle, and that will magnify the returns on your lifestyle-change investment. If you get into a habit of doing this, your body will spend no less than 12 hours a day burning fat and 12 hours a day burning the food you eat. The only difference between the different diets of food is whether you want to have a heavy workout or you want to have a light workout. That will depend on the extent of your meal.

Daily Strategy

Your daily strategy starts immediately after your induction week. You ended your induction week with a 3 hour fast, so instead of a 12-hour window, you have an 8-hour window. That's not too bad a difference. In this window, you should think about how many meals you want to have. As time goes by, you can adjust this, and I don't want to enforce my preferred number of meals into this because I know there are many people with different metabolic profiles, so some of you may optimize your window with multiple small meals, and some of you may optimize with just three large meals. Whichever you choose, it must follow:

1.The intensity of the meals must be on a descending profile - that means your second meal of the window must be the largest, followed by something slightly less, then a lesser, and finally, your last meal in the window should be the smallest of all.
2.Break the fast with an appetizer or a protein shake, or even BCAA after a light workout.
3.Have a heavy workout before your heavy meal.
4.Have the heaviest meal after the workout.
5.Have the lightest meal before closing the eating window.

Here is what happens when you do this.
1. You convert fat to muscle, and I am not talking about becoming chiseled and cut. I am talking about lean and toned.
2. When you have more muscle mass, it requires more energy to support - which allows you to eat more and burn more fat.

3. The more fat you burn, the more energy you have coursing through you, and the more lean energy you send to your brain. Remember, your brain works better with energy derived from fat - you are sharper and more agile with quicker response times and astute observation.

4. When you start your day with a boost to the metabolism, you burn energy all day, so you have set yourself on an automatic path to consistent fuel conversion.

Daily Schedule A

There are two possible schedules you can use to get you started. This is the first one, and it applies to those with intense workouts in the first part of their day. You can create your own schedule after you are more familiar with your body's responses, and you can fine-tune it from there. For now, this will get you started.

This works well if you are in the office and have a gym close by.

12 noon Light workout

12.15 Breakfast with a light shake or protein, or BCAA followed by a workout until 1 pm

1 pm Largest Meal of the day

8 pm Window Closes

Between 1 pm and 8 pm, you can have as many meals as you want, but they must be in decreasing quantity over time, with the smallest happening before 8 pm.

Daily Schedule B

12 noon Light workout

12.15 breakfast with light shake and appetizers. Wait 20 minutes and go on to the heaviest meal of the day.

4 pm Second meal of the day

7 pm Third meal of the day.

8 pm Window Closes

Between these schedules, the first is for those who want to supplement their fasting with a workout (which I highly recommend); the second is for those who have a smaller workout to get your juices flowing and then go on to the meal.

There are two other variants you can try. You just have to remember the idea is that you switch back and forth between metabolic fuel sources. By fasting for twelve hours and having an eating window for eight hours, you are promoting a better switching rate between fuel sources, and that promotes a more balanced lifestyle.

The other thing you must remember is that while you are fasting, you must keep active. You must be at work, at play, at the gym, or up and about. The last thing you want to do is do nothing. Doing nothing will get you to think of snacking and food, and it slows down your metabolism. When you get up and move about, it keeps the flow and keeps your mind off food. Working includes reading, studying, and office work. It doesn't just mean physical work. However, if you are sitting all day at work, get up and move about to keep the circulation going.

CHAPTER EIGHTEEN: ADDITIONAL VARIATIONS OF FEASTING-FASTING

There are other variants of the feasting-fasting schedule you can try besides the first two above. The main difference is that the feeding phase and the workout sessions do not coincide. It is a little heavier for those who are not used to it, but it works well at burning weight and building muscle tone. The reason this one actually works better is that the metabolic state you are in after the workout burns fatter than if it were in a sedated state. To accomplish this, follow this routine:

Variation A

6 am Pre-Workout Routine

6.10 Supplement intake (BCAA - 10 grams) this does not count as eating

6.15 Heavy workout for 60 minutes

8 am BCAA - 10 grams

10 am BCAA 10 Grams

Noon - First main meal of the day marking the start of the Eating Window

7 - 8 pm - Last meal of the day

Between noon and 8 pm, you can have as many meals as you would like, as long as you remember they should be decreasing in quantity.

Variation B

5 am Last meal in the Eating Window

6 am Pre-Workout Routine and start of the Fasting phase

6.10 Supplement intake (BCAA - 10 grams); this does not count toward the Eating Window

6.15 Heavy workout for 60 minutes

8 am BCAA - 10 grams

10 am BCAA 10 Grams

8.30 pm Lite appetizers (Fasting Window)

8.45 Lite workout

9.30 pm First heavy meal

10 pm Second heave meal followed by sleep

5 am Wake up and a light meal before fasting window

This will allow you to spend your waking hours fasting and constantly burning fat, and staying active. If you start to lose excess weight, then increase your intake during the eating widow - do not shorten the fasting cycle.

CHAPTER NINETEEN: THE CHALLENGE OF INTERMITTENT FASTING

If you are doing this and you are past the first week, you are probably adhering to the intermittent fasting lifestyle. The hardest part of fasting is the mindset we bring to the table. You are not the only one. Millions of people come to the dinner table with everything except nutrition on their minds. They come to the table for a family reunion. They come for pleasure in the taste and decoration of the food. They come for the habit yet don't realize it. They come to fulfill their obligation to eat, even when they are not hungry.

The most important aspect of coming to the table is for you to think you are coming there for nutrition. Think about food as just a way to fuel and repair your body. It may be one of the most boring ways to see things, but that is what you are doing. It's time to have a food revolution and stop thinking about food as a source of pleasure and think of food as a source of life. Eating is part of the circle of life, and eating allows us to go into the world to be more than we currently even think about.

Mindful Eating

At the core of Intermittent Fasting is a concept that most of us are not aware of until we realize our state when we eat. We are usually in a rush to have a meal, or we are busy doing something else. It is a source of entertainment and a source of pleasure. None of this actually aids in eating healthy.

When you practice intermittent fasting, you should shift how you see your meal and practice mindful eating.

Mindful eating is about being one with your food and focusing on the eating process, rather than just stuffing yourself while you are doing something else. When you eat just twice a day, once in the morning and once in the afternoon, you should spend no more than 20 - 30 minutes consuming your food. Do it in silence and absorb the experience.

This is not so much about having fun with your food, but it's a process of getting intimate with your nutrition. Mindful eating will change your life when you do it with Intermittent Fasting. You will find your body adapts to the changes in your habits and in the changes to the lack of pleasure motives in the act of nutrition consumption.

Have Fun

Having fun is not a bad thing. Many helpful things in life will give you pleasure, but you shouldn't look at all these things for pleasure for pleasure's sake. Driving to work every day is a mindful experience while you pay attention to your vehicle and the other drivers on the road. You pay attention to your driving and your route to the destination. But just because you love racing cars on the weekend doesn't mean you must drive fast on the road. Eating is about eating; having fun is about entertainment. Sometimes, eating can be about fun, but that is the exception, not the norm.

The power of intermittent fasting is it shifts your focus and your habits away from something that is unnatural and unhealthy. It takes your body's dependence on repeated introduction to food and puts it where it belongs, on the dependence on stored resources. It also puts you in control over the kinds of food and increases your reliance on a healthy appetite. The power of intermittent fasting is that it is a liberalizing endeavor that allows you to take control of your life.

Junk Food

The term is used in this book with no sense of exaggeration. Junk food is junk. They are loaded with calories and mind-altering compounds that give you a feeling of euphoria while decreasing your health and altering your preference from things that are healthy to things that are addictive.

Why do I keep emphasizing eating healthy and avoiding processed food? Because you can actually eat crap food and lose weight while doing intermittent fasting. This is not a permanent solution. You might feel sharp and healthy as you are losing your excess fat, but your body will break at some point.

CHAPTER TWENTY: MENTAL FRAMEWORK

Once you have your initial experience of the Intermittent Fast and you are getting comfortable with it, you must begin cleansing your mind. We do this with mindfulness achieved through breathing exercises. Wait, what, you might say? What does cleansing the mind has to do with intermittent fasting? It is all about lifestyle changes. Eating like your body is meant to eat is just one part of the equation. So, this is why we next look into some mindful practices I have found to be useful when combined with fasting.

Stage 1 Breathing Exercise

The first stage, exercise, initiates you into a sequence of breathing and mindfulness exercises. There are four stages you will go through before you begin to see the effects that will astonish you.

The beginning of Stage 1 is simple. Find a spot you are comfortable with. Close your eyes. You have no other tasks to accomplish. When you do this with your eyes closed, it will seem as though you are watching from a point between your two eyes, just above the bridge of your nose in the middle of your forehead. It will only seem like this. Identify this as the seat of your inner Self.

Once you close your eyes, watch your breathing. That's all you need to do. Remember to place all other distractions on hold. When you sit down and watch your breathing, count how long it takes to inhale. 1 Mississippi ... 2 Mississippi... 3 Mississippi... until your breath reaches the end of its natural cycle and prepares to exhale. Remember, you are only watching, not controlling. So, whatever rhythm of breathing that is currently a part of you is what you are watching. Do not try to change it to inhale deeply or exhale fully. Breath naturally.

When you do this, you will note the number of seconds it takes to inhale. Then count the time it takes to exhale. The time it takes to exhale might be the same time as the inhale, and for now, that does not matter. Keep doing this for 10 minutes in the beginning. When you progress, you can extend your exhalation compared to inhalation and extend your breathing to 15-20 minutes.

When done, open your eyes and relax in the same position, and slowly let the rest of life enter your conscious observation. Listen to each sound as it enters your consciousness. Then open your eyes and let the information flood you.

As you become aware of your surroundings, remember only what you must. Because you have just realized that, when you are flooded with information, your mind can only pay partial attention to any one thing.

When you repeat this every day for a week, you will do two things: you will slow down your rhythm, and you will peel away whatever stress you are facing, even if you didn't know you had any. But this is just the first part. To understand nature, slowing down is a major part of success.

Stage 2 Controlled Breathing

The second part is when you begin to control your breathing to match the inhale and exhale times. By matching the times, you are intentionally controlling your breathing. But do not jump to this step right away. You must take it slowly. The chances are that you are like 99% of people around the world and your breathing techniques are wrong. If you learned to breathe right from a young age, your diaphragm would be strong, and you can control your tempo well.

While breathing, you should slowly realize, aside from the better breathing habits and the calming of your mind, your extremities begin to tingle. It just means that your pulse oxygen level is going up. You are sending more oxygen to the rest of your body, and it is literally waking up.

With this simple exercise, and without too much effort, you have begun to cleanse your body and oxidize much of the gaseous toxins that are present. By doing the weekly water fast, you have also cleansed your gut, and by doing that, you have improved the quality of your blood. With the increased blood quality and the increased breathing, oxygen will be flowing in abundance, and your cells will rejuvenate themselves. The increased Vitamin C from the fruits you are now taking in replacement of the junk food is also helping your immune system to boost its performance.

Stage 3 Visualize Your Distractions
The third stage of meditation will help you quit the habit of eating and get you on the road to health. The third stage is also rather simple, and you need only to extend the time you take away for meditation.

The idea is to visualize your distractions, and eating is a distraction. When you get to this stage, you are acknowledging your distractions but do not participate in them. You will find your thoughts have a mind of their own. Those thoughts are beyond yourself, and you are separating yourself from random fragments of thought. Don't worry - everybody has them.

When watching your breathing, you will realize you can monitor everything that goes on about you. The same thing is now expanded when you look at not just what you are doing with your breath but also what you are doing within your mind. The thoughts you have will be more visible to your mind's eye, and you can watch them go by without interacting with them.

The benefit of this third stage is that you are becoming the master of your mind, so you can be less stressed in many situations. To reap the benefits, keep going and never stop the daily meditation routine and the weekly fasting.

The mindfulness exercises you have been practicing allow you to remember one salient truth that the past and the future do not matter, and what matters is the moment. Being mindful is about being in the moment. Being in the moment is the most important thing in the world when trying to do anything in this world.

Stage 4 Instantaneous Focus

When you get to this stage, the idea is to control your breathing at the drop of a dime - to control what your mind is doing at the drop of a dime - to control where you are in a moment. And once you can do that, you have reached the pinnacle of simple meditation. There is no need to visualize anything. Your breath is the most powerful thing in the world. Between your mind and your breath, there is almost nothing you cannot cure. In stage four, it is time to move your meditation to other parts of your life. Wherever you are, pay full attention to what you are doing.

Wherever you are, make sure you are in the moment, especially when eating. Whether you are on the bus, on a plane, be mindful. Being mindful is not about being withdrawn. You are fully aware of all that is happening around you. You are not participating, but you are watching.

Meditation has a multi-dimensional effect on everyone. It is one of the best ways to get in touch with what is going on inside you. With mindfulness exercises and breathing exercises, one benefit you will experience is that your body will tell you what it needs. This will cause you to get visions of what is necessary and what you must eat. It will be the way your body tells you what it needs from a nutritional standpoint. When you combine Intermittent Fasting with meditation and mindfulness, you get in touch with your body and understand what your body wants.

Your mental health and framework is an important aspect of all things you do, even the way you think about the way you eat. When you embark on a quest for a healthier life and a more finely tuned body, mindfulness in all that you do will only take you to higher accomplishments. Being able to counter the temptation cultivated from decades of incorrect eating patterns is better handled with meditation and mindfulness.

If you feel you have appreciated my effort, I kindly ask you to leave a (positive) review! It will help me to create something new and useful for your interest: =)

M.T